YOUR KNOWLEDGE HAS VALUE

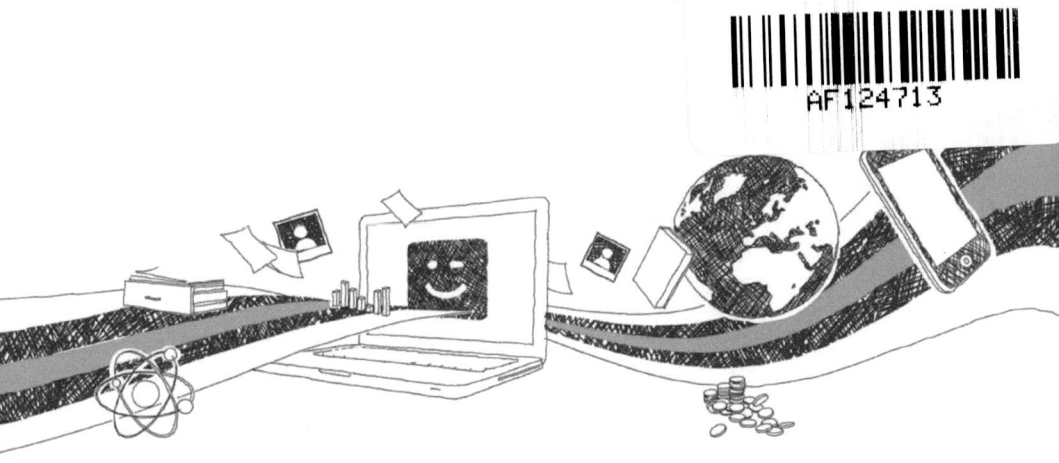

- We will publish your bachelor's and master's thesis, essays and papers

- Your own eBook and book - sold worldwide in all relevant shops

- Earn money with each sale

Upload your text at www.GRIN.com
and publish for free

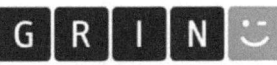

Bibliographic information published by the German National Library:

The German National Library lists this publication in the National Bibliography; detailed bibliographic data are available on the Internet at http://dnb.dnb.de .

Imprint:

Copyright © 2018 GRIN Verlag
Print and binding: Books on Demand GmbH, Norderstedt Germany
ISBN: 9783668877030

This book at GRIN:

https://www.grin.com/document/454127

Janos Talaber

How Can Paramedics be Involved Efficiently in Medical Care at Emergency Hospital Units?

A Legal Overview Concerning the UK, the USA, Canada and Hungary

GRIN Verlag

GRIN - Your knowledge has value

Since its foundation in 1998, GRIN has specialized in publishing academic texts by students, college teachers and other academics as e-book and printed book. The website www.grin.com is an ideal platform for presenting term papers, final papers, scientific essays, dissertations and specialist books.

Visit us on the internet:

http://www.grin.com/

http://www.facebook.com/grincom

http://www.twitter.com/grin_com

University of Hertfordshire
Hatfield, UK

János Talabér:

Off-board Paramedics – Paramedics in Hospital Emergency Rooms

(A Legal Overview Concerning the UK, the USA, Canada, and Hungary)

Paramedic, Bsc.

TABLE OF CONTENTS

.

I Introduction

The purpose of this short study, does not matter what we call it now, is to highlight the legal possibilities of employing paramedics off-board, which means, we would like to focus on the possible options to involve them into medical care at emergency hospital units. It is obvious that we lack medical doctors, nurses and other high trained staff not only in hospital wards, but also in pre-hospital emergency care. To overlap this lack and hiatus, it was several times noted in Hungary that as for competency reasons, the closest medical staff to be involved in emergency medical treatments is the paramedics. We have been dealing with medical law for more than a decade, and have been on board as paramedics (EMTs) for more than two decades now. The accurate scopes of Paramedics, competency and other conditions vary differently in the World, therefore there is not a consequent and primarily accepted competency. However, serving the streets and responding to dispatches is pretty much similar in all over the World, therefore, the main streams are almost totally related.

Throughout this document we will see the scopes and competencies as well as the education strategies of paramedic trainings in Canada, the USA and within the European Union.

II The scope of Paramedic Science in the USA and Canada

A paramedic is a healthcare professional, providing pre-hospital assessment and medical care to people with acute illnesses or injuries. In Canada and the USA, the title paramedic generally refers to those who work on land ambulances or air ambulances providing paramedic services. More and more paramedics in the USA and Canada are increasingly being utilized in emergency rooms by providing patient care in collaboration with physicians, physician assistants, nurse practitioners, registered nurses, registered practical nurses and registered respiratory therapists. Increasingly in Canada, paramedics are actively pursuing self-regulation.[1]

On the other hand, the Advanced Paramedic in Ireland, for instance, is principally engaged in responding to patients who access the 999/112 service for emergency medical assistance and can provide advanced life support. This includes the skills listed for Paramedic and the use of an endotracheal tube, intravenous cannulation, manual defibrillation, thrombolysis, needle thoracocentesis, needle cricothyrotomy and urinary catheterization.[2] Paramedic education, or the study of paramedicine in Canada or in the States, is an intensive academic program of formal theory and clinical experience which varies from province to province. For example, the primary care paramedic program may be three months in class with 12 days on the ambulance for precepting, or a two year diploma or four year degree in primary care paramedicine in other universities. Training as an advanced care paramedic requires that the student be first registered as a primary care paramedic. Eligibility for this training varies from immediate entry following a registration to a mandatory period of experience working as a paramedic usually one to three years. The length of time required to complete paramedic training also varies between provinces, and it is generally inversely related to the length of time required to have completed the prerequisite training.[3] Shorter (around one year) programs build upon the education already learned in a two-year paramedic training program, while longer (typically up to two years) college programs typically cater to paramedics who graduated from shorter programs

Therefore, while there is continual debate on the merits of longer or shorter paramedic programs (often centered around teaching philosophy), in common, ACPs across Canada and the USA will generally have completed approximately three years of intensive formal education,

---

[1]Talabér j., , Kompetenciák a sürgősségi betegellátásban , Előadás: Szeged, MRT Kongresszus, 2007. szeptember 15.

[2] http://ec.europa.eu/growth/tools-databases/regprof/index.cfm?action=regprof&id_regprof=26427

[3] Göbl G. Oxiológia, Medicina, Budapest, 2006.

4

inclusive of didactic study and clinical placements. There are ASS (Associate Bachelor) degrees of advanced EMT cares, Bachelor degrees (BSc), and also Masters degrees in APN (Advanced Practice Nurse).

There are two Bachelor of Health Science in paramedicine degrees currently available in Canada and in the USA, are becoming the standard of paramedic education as the profession progresses at the Primary Care Paramedic entry level. This would be comparable to when nursing moved from the college based program to the collaborative or university based program in Canada. These programs are often offered through partnerships between Canadian universities and colleges, blending vocational training with higher education. (eg. EMT-Advanced and Paramedic BSc).

Paramedic degrees were probably first created overseas and in the UK, therefore in the European Community, this education was for long ignored. After the Second World War it came into a primary focus, since there was a very severe lack of medical doctors, and also the view and aspect of primary medical treatment had changed. It became absolutely obvious that no medical doctor degree would be needed for primary medical cares, hence a good trained nurse or a paramedic (at that time ambulance nurse) could intervene if it was needed.[4]

The accreditation of paramedic educational programs in Canada also varies from province to province. The Canadian Medical Association's Committee on Conjoint Accreditation offers the most comprehensive and best known system of national accreditation.[5] Their accreditation model is an independent body, and draws from The "National Occupational Competency

[4]Talabér j., "Mentő protokoll? - eljárásrend szemle jogász szemmel"., MSOTKE Konferencia, Budapest, 2015. november 12-15.

Profile" as the benchmark document that details the knowledge, skills and abilities outcomes that must be possessed by practitioners of each respective level of paramedic practice.

In Canada the scope of practice of paramedics is described by the National Occupational Competency Profile (NOCP) for Paramedics document developed by the Paramedic Association of Canada with financial support from the Government of Canada. The NOCP outlines four provider levels: Emergency Medical Responder (EMR), Primary Care Paramedic (PCP), Advanced Care Paramedic (ACP), and Critical Care Paramedic (CCP)

III Provincial variations on the National Occupational Competency Profile[5]

Of considerable relevance to understanding the nature of Canadian paramedic practice, the reader must appreciate the considerable degree of inter-provincial variation. Although a national consensus (by way of the National Occupational Competency Profile) identifies certain knowledge, skills, and abilities as being most synonymous with a given level of paramedic practice, each province retains ultimate authority in legislating the actual administration and delivery of emergency medical services within its own borders. For this reason, any discussion of *paramedic practice* in Canada is necessarily broad, and general. Specific regulatory frameworks and questions related to paramedic practice can only definitively be answered by consulting relevant provincial legislation, although provincial paramedic associations may often offer a simpler overview of this topic when it is restricted to a province-by-province basis.

Regulatory frameworks vary from province to province, and include direct government regulation (such as Ontario's method of credentialing its practitioners with the title of A-EMCA, or Advanced Emergency Medical Care Attendant) to professional self-regulating bodies, such as the Alberta College of Paramedics. Though the title of paramedic is a generic description of

---

[5] https://en.wikipedia.org/wiki/Paramedics_in_the_United_States

a category of practitioners, provincial variability in regulatory methods accounts for ongoing differences in actual titles that are ascribed to different levels of practitioners. For example, the province of British Columbia is the only province that uses the title "Infant Transport Team Paramedic", or 'ITT Paramedic' for PARAMEDICs who have received additional critical care training for pediatric, neonatal, and high risk obstetric emergencies.[8] All provinces, however, have moved to standard titles, or have at least recognized the NOCP document as a benchmark document to permit inter-provincial labor mobility of practitioners, regardless of how titles are specifically regulated within their own provincial systems.

IV Special types of Paramedics in the USA[6]

Training for specialization as a paramedic is most often provided by employers who select paramedics that have gone through an internal competition. There are very few specialization education programs open to the public currently. An exception being STARS Critical Care and Transport Medicine Academy, offered jointly by STARS Air Ambulance and the University of Calgary. Most specializations require the applicant to already be an experienced advanced care paramedic.

A. Critical care paramedic

Critical care paramedics' (CCP) expertise focus on critical and ICU level care, stabilizing and transporting patients from smaller hospitals with less available resources to tertiary care, and regional medical programs in to other hospitals that can provide a higher level of care. CCPs generally work with an ACP, registered nurse, physician, or another CCP. Sometimes ad hoc teams, with multiple practitioners (RTs, emergency physicians, surgeons, etc.) are assembled for certain patients.

---

[6] "Nationwide Directory of Paramedic Schools". Retrieved 2008-11-07.

CCPs are able to provide all of the care that PARAMEDICs and ACPs provide. In addition to this they are trained for other skills such as medication infusion pumps, mechanical ventilation and arterial line monitoring. CCPs often work in fixed and rotary wing aircraft when the weather permits and staff are available, but systems such as the Toronto EMS Critical Care Transport Program work in land ambulances. ORNGE Transport operates both land and aircraft in Ontario. In British Columbia, CCP's work primarily in aircraft with a dedicated Critical Care Transport crew in several cities for long-distance/high acuity transfers and as regular CCP street crews who may do major trauma calls or, performs medevacs, when necessary. Across the prairies, rotary wing aircraft is used to reach many in isolated communities and traumatic situations for faster response time than by ground ambulance. In Saskatchewan they also use fixed wing air ambulances. The service, called Lifeguard, can respond a greater distance and to more northern communities than STARS. Sask air ambulance service was the first non-military air ambulance service in the world.[14] These air ambulances are crewed by Flight Nurses and CCPs.

B. Tactical paramedic

Tactical paramedics are specialized paramedics who undergo additional training to allow them to perform their usual task in a high risk and dangerous scenario. Some are trained to handle weapons, repel from buildings and other skills needed to work alongside tactical police units. These paramedics are required to wear protective gear but are unarmed.

C. Occupational health paramedic

Occupational health paramedics work closely with occupational physicians and nurses to help with pre-employment screening, medical surveillance programs and clinical testing for companies.

D. Community paramedic

The newest level/role for paramedics in Canada and in the USA, community paramedics work in clinics, hospitals, and in patient's homes. They provide immediate or scheduled primary, urgent and specialized healthcare to vulnerable patient populations by collaborating with other healthcare providers, conducting assessments, treating, and doing/ordering tests.[7] Diagnostics provided by Community Paramedics: Specimen collection (blood, urine, swabs), 12/15 lead ECGs, vital signs (temperature, blood glucose, SPO2, side stream CO2, BP), and facilitate transports for diagnostic imaging. Treatments provided by Community Paramedics: CVC & IV rehydration, blood transfusions, urinary catheterization, wound closure & care (tissue adhesive, sutures, dressings), oxygen and nebulizer therapy, IV/SQ/IM/PO/PORT/PICC medication administration (including IV antibiotics), and coordination of community services.

E. Incident response paramedic

A type of specialization in Al Metro areas, IRPs receive intensive training, including toxicology, hazmat chemistry, National Fire Protection Association hazmat awareness and operations certifications, as well as three weeks of CBRNE training, antidote, medical countermeasures, MCI and, protective equipment training.

For day-to-day operations, IRPs respond to hazmat- and toxicology-related incidents. They carry a wider range of medications than advanced care paramedics and more protective

---

[7] "National EMS Scope of Practice" (PDF). Retrieved 2012-11-11.

equipment, allowing them to better treat poisonings/overdoses and work closely with firefighters and hazmat technicians.

F. Paramedic specialist

ACPs and CCPs in British Columbia that provide on-scene technical support for high-risk situations, mass and complex patient events as well as telephone support to paramedics and patients. Typically work in solo response vehicles in Metro areas or in dispatch centres.

G. Infant transport team paramedic

Only a designation in British Columbia, ITT paramedics are specially trained ALS paramedics who undergo extra training to provide emergency medical care for BC pediatric, neo-natal and high-risk obstetrics patients while en route to specialized care units in hospitals throughout British Columbia, the Yukon Territories, other parts of Canada and the United States as required.

V. Laws for Paramedics in the UK[8]

The legal system in place within the UK can be broadly divided into two main branches: criminal law and civil law. Table 1.1 details the differences and similarities between these two areas. Paramedics are subject to the same legislation as any other individual in the UK, and are specifically named in practice notes for particular legislation such as the Mental Capacity Act 2005. In practice, the majority of legislation that impacts on the day-to-day work of the paramedic is dealt with by the paramedic's employing authority. Health and safety, data protection, drugs regulation, medical equipment safety, and human rights are all areas that are legislated and put in place by employers. Paramedics as individuals are more likely to fall foul of the civil side of the law if they either lack competence or engage in behavior which could be

---

[8] V.Clarke, G.Harris, S. Cowland (eds), Ethics and Laws For Paramedics, London, 2009.

considered as misconduct. This will be discussed under the heading of professional regulation. A third branch of the legal system is that of the coroner's inquest. Threats of 'explain it to the coroner' have historically been used to encourage student paramedics to do the right thing when treating patients and when completing records, often portraying the coroner as someone to be feared. This is simply not the case. The role of the coroner in relation to deceased individuals is to establish facts. There are four main facts that the coroner must establish: the identity of the deceased; the place of death; the time of death; how the deceased came by their death. Coroners are usually lawyers with specialist training, with only about 25 per cent being medical doctors with a legal qualification. The coroner's inquest follows an inquisitorial process which aims only to establish the facts, as opposed to criminal and civil cases which follow an adversarial process with one side trying to prove that their case is more just than their opponents. Paramedics may be called upon to provide written witness statements of fact to the coroner and any patient report records that they have completed may also be subjected to scrutiny. Moreover, in some cases where further clarification is needed, the paramedic may be required to give evidence at a coroner's inquest. Once the paramedic has answered any of the coroner's questions, the coroner may invite any interested parties to question the paramedic. This means that relatives of the deceased, or their representatives, may ask the paramedic questions. This can be a difficult and uncomfortable experience for the paramedic concerned, but it often goes a long way to giving bereaved relatives a greater understanding of what happened to their loved one. In order to make such experiences as pain free as possible, it is vital that the paramedic thoroughly documents all details for all the calls that they attend.[9]

---

[9] https://www.mheducation.co.uk/openup/chapters/9780335243877.pdf

VI.   The history and structure of ambulance care in Hungary

As it is still today, The National Ambulance Service (NAS) is the largest medical and ambulance institution of Hungary which have carried out rescue and patient transport duties since nearly seventy years. Today it has more than 7,500 employees.

The history of the Hungarian organized ambulance system dates back to the last third of the 19th century in our country. In addition, the predecessors of NAS were the Budapest Volunteer Ambulance Association, founded in 1887, and the Counties and Cities Ambulance Association, founded in 1926, which was operated a nation-wide ambulance station network. Moreover, founded with infrastructural background and knowledge gathered through generations, the new country wide competent institution, NAS is the guarantee of the history and developing of rescuing of the past 129 years. Furthermore, one of the most telling example is that in the year of the nationalization of rescue, in 1948, the Counties and Cities Ambulance Association provided the infrastructure and the personnel for the new organization, also the Budapest Volunteer Ambulance Association ensured the medical professional background.[10] The modernization of the ambulance is steadily on-going. Our ambulance service developed further in the way of more centralized structure, has been built up a kind of hierarchical form. Accordingly, its operation is incomparable. For today, the National Ambulance Service has tripled the number of its ambulance stations, twenty-fold manpower and the number of cars has increased six-fold.

---

[10] http://www.mentomuzeum.hu/eng/about-nas

A. Institutional structure

As to ensure more efficient operation, the National Ambulance Service established the county rescue organizations in county seats around the mid-sixties managed by the local chief medical officers, whereas the director and professional administrative departments decided technical and organizational matters. In the beginning, their decisions were binding on all county rescue organizations, and arrive in the form of circulars.

The year 2005 brought changes in the structure when the NAS formed the regional ambulance organizations, which have taken over the role of the county rescue organizations. Seven regions were established:

- Middle Hungary (Regional Ambulance Organization - RAO) headquartered in Budapest called KMR (the main headquarter)
- Central Transdanubia RAO headquartered in Veszprém;
- Western Transdanubia RAO headquartered in Szombathely;
- Southern Transdanubia RAO headquartered in Pécs;
- Southern Great Plain RAO headquartered in Szeged;
- Northern Great Plain RAO headquartered in Debrecen;
- Northern Hungary RAO headquartered in Miskolc.

In these regions, officers, paramedics and local chief medical doctors perform their duties in accordance with the former governing mechanism.

B. Ambulance station network

In the very beginning, eg.in the year of the founding National Ambulance Service, the Hungarian ambulance station network consisted of 76 stations. However, during the next twenty years and also the 1980s, the development was ongoing. Today, the NAS has 254 ambulance stations, and other two (one in Pest county) are now being built at the time of our writing this essay. We distinguish three categories of ambulance stations (A, B, C,) by the number and types of ambulance vehicles. The number of vehicles functioning every day is 782 out of 1,065 vehicles. This means we are in great lack of medical experts, just as in all parts of Europe. [11]Also, alternative (eg. charity) ambulance services could also be involved in rescue if they fulfill the legal requirements. [12] On the other hand, the rescue controlling is an integral part of ambulance work, then the NAS manages the whole vehicles fleet along unified professional principles from 19 rescue controlling call centers throughout with a nation-wide coverage of telecommunications apparatus. The new rescue call centers and new number is being introduced, with uncertain and questionable remarks. However, the ambulance units take 38 up to 40 million kilometers on roads in Hungary per year. 7500 employees work in the National Ambulance Service, who carry out more than one million tasks a year.

VII. Act 18/2016 Hungarian Competency Act of Health Care Workers[13]

In accordance with the 2011 CCIV National Higher Education Act (3) (b) of the Hungarian Government ordered the following act: general characteristics and competences describing the level of education obtainable in higher education.

A. About the Act

Annex 2 sets out the characteristics of a common module for all higher education professional training and in tertiary education and the training and output requirements for higher education vocational training courses. Moreover, Annex 3 specifies the training and output requirements for higher education undergraduate courses per training area. Whereas, Annex 4 sets out the

---

[11] http://statinfo.ksh.hu/Statinfo/haViewer.jsp

[12] www.dabasmok.hu

[13] see also: TALABÉR J., Az ellátók és ellátottak jogai és kötelezettségei, Pusztaföldvár, Egészség Napok Továbbképzés sorozat, 2018. május 23.

14

training and output requirements of the higher education masters programs per training area, with the exception of teacher training courses, Annex 5 sets out the requirements for joint training of Hungarian and foreign higher education institutions.

Following this, Annex 6 sets out the training and output requirements of the courses of the subject of the subject, whereas Section 12 In the core and master courses and in higher education vocational competences, out of which the competences to be acquired must include the knowledge of computer literacy, the training of digital training contents corresponding to vocational and professional education and training, as well as the basics of health promotion and sustainable development including environmental, accident, work - and basic consumer protection.

In addition, Section 3 notes that if the training and output requirements of vocational education and training in tertiary education do not differ from the special marks that distinguish the training, the training may be organized as full-time and part-time as defined in its curriculum and as distance education. (- it is how learning procedure could be carried out in the UK and USA as well).[14] Furthermore, training and output requirements, as defined by this Regulation, shall be applied in full-time and part-time and in distance learning as well as undergraduate and master training and higher education vocational training. Vocational (eg. professional) training in higher education may be awarded to a higher education qualification who possesses the following knowledge, skills, attitudes, autonomy and responsibility competencies as it follows.

---

[14]*TALABÉR J., Off-board mentőtiszt - jogszerűen a sürgősségin és az orvosi ügyeleten? , MSOTKE, 2018. (poszter), Siófok.*

B. General skills

a. Knowledge
- Provides general and specific theoretical and practical knowledge related to a particular field;

- His theoretical and practical knowledge is organized into a system.

- Familiarize knowledge and problem-solving methods with core theories.

- Provides a solid knowledge of the practical methods and tools required for long-term and high-level education in that profession.

- Knows the vocabulary of the field in mother tongue and has at least one foreign language level basic knowledge of languages.[15]

- Knows the values of his profession in the context of contemporary culture.

b. Abilities
- Providing the appropriate job qualification.

- Designing and solving the tasks of the given profession by selecting the necessary methods and tools, with its unique and complex application.

- Communicating professionally through mother-tongue and foreign-language communication skills.

- Developing knowledge and applying it to various methods of acquiring knowledge, self-development and using the most up-to-date information and communication tools.

- Recognize the relationship between personal development and service of the public good.

---

[15] Please note that since the year 2010 no degrees could be awarded without the recipients having the intermediate certificate of foreign language. Therefore, those graduating after 2010 can be expected to speak at least one foreign language fluently.

c. Attitude

- Open to the new achievements and innovations of this field, it seeks to understand, understand and apply it.

- Seeking continuous self-education.

- Self-critical about his own work.

- Accepts and credibly conveys the social role and values of his profession.

- Prepared for unexpected life situations, makes decision with full regard to the laws and ethical norms.

- Open to professional cooperation with professionals who work in other fields.

d. Autonomy and Responsibility

- Performs your work independently, with continuous self-checking.

- Takes responsibility for the work, results and failures of his own and the professional team he leads.

- Has a level of responsibility and reflects on the consequences of its own activity.

Characteristics of the level of education available in the initial training: undergraduate students can acquire a Bachelor's Degree who has the following knowledge, skills, attitudes, autonomy and responsibility competencies (extra competencies for a Bsc).

a) knowledge

- Comprehensively understands the basic facts, directions, and boundaries of the subject area of the given field of study.

- Knows the most important relationships, theories, and the concepts that make up for them.

- Familiarizes knowledge and problem-solving methods with core theories.

- Possesses the range of knowledge required to enter a Master's Degree in a particular field and other field of study.
- Comprehensively understands the legal regulations related to his field of expertise, ethical norms.
- Possesses the knowledge, the abilities and attitudes that engage the profession in a certain circle of civic literacy.

b) Abilities

- Provides the appropriate job qualification.
- Performs the basic analysis of the disciplines that make up the knowledge system of its field of expertise, synthetic formulation and adequate evaluation of the relationships.
- Applies the procedures, key theories, and related terminology when executing its tasks.
- Understands and uses the online and printed literature in its field of expertise in Hungarian and foreign languages, with the knowledge of effective information retrieval and processing for its field of expertise.
- Understands or interprets coherent texts, as well as texts, tables, data series, visual texts, moving images, stills, maps, diagrams, as well as visual signs, typographic tools, icons.
- Identifies routine professional problems, reveals and formulates the conceptual and practical background needed to solve them, solves them by practicing standard operations.
- Plans and organizes own learning, using the widest range of available resources.
- At workplace, manages resources by using your professional skills.

c) Attitude

- Entrusts and credibly represents the social role of the profession, its fundamental relation to the world.

- Open to profession is the authentic mediation and transfer of the basic features of its comprehensive thinking and practical operation.

- Open to the knowledge, acceptance and authentication of professional, technological development and innovation in its field.

- Strives to make self-education one of the tools of achieving its professional goals.

- Takes its decision with full regard to the laws and ethical norms in a complex approach or unexpected decision situations.

- Strives to solve problems in cooperation with others.

- Interprets continuous personal learning in the service of the public good.

d) Autonomy and Responsibility

- In the case of unexpected decision-making situations, he also performs self-conceptualization of comprehensive, grounded professional issues and elaboration of the given resources.

- Takes on the basis of professional guidance the elaboration of comprehensive and specialized professional issues and the elaboration of resources based on specific sources.

- Works independently on critical evaluation and continuous correction of its activity.

- Responsible for developing and explaining professional views.

- Assumes the underlying views of his or her field of expertise.

- Develops new skills through independent continuing education or organized training

C. Common Competencies in Nursing and Patient Treating Professionals (7.1.1.)

a) knowledge

- Knows the organization's structure, its legality, the function of the various components, the biochemical regulatory and metabolic processes in detail.

- Knows the structure structures of the organ systems, the microscopic and macroscopic structure of the organ systems, the surface structures of the formulas, the physiological and abnormal functioning of the organism, knows their regulation and the pathogenesis of pathological processes in the body

- Familiar with the typical macroscopic and microscopic structural changes of the most common diseases.

- Familiar with the main diagnostic methods and principles of operation.

- Familiar with the specifics of the therapeutic environment, the effects, the range of indications and the course of implementation of different bed types, bed positions, postures, comfort devices, mobilization devices and procedures.

- Knows the anatomical and physiological basis of analgesics and the various analgesics.

- Knows the basics of meeting physiological needs.

- Knows the types and methodologies of healthcare documentation.

- Familiar with the subject, tasks, distribution, methods, basic concepts of occupational health and prevention, the effects of the environment on humans, and details of public health epidemiology.

- Knows in detail the subject of microbiology, its functions, its distribution, the distribution of microbes and all the features that are relevant to the development of infections.

- Knows the possibilities of detection and destruction of microorganisms, such as pathologies, sampling rules, sampling methods.
- Knows the concepts of asepsis-antisepsis, nosocomialis surveillance, the essence and course of selective waste collection.
- Knows the range of indications of the measurement of vital parameters, the procedure of evaluating the interventions and the results obtained (including mantle and core respiration, facial types, type of breath sample, pulse rate and quality, pulse defect, noninvasive measurement of arterial blood pressure) (including the applicable tools, procedures, and indicative routines).
- Knows the range of indications of the measurement of vital parameters, the procedure of evaluating the interventions and the results obtained (including mantle and core respiration, facial types, type of breath sample, pulse rate and quality, pulse defect, noninvasive measurement of arterial blood pressure) (including the applicable tools, procedures, and indicative routines).
- Determines in detail the basic elements, forms, directions, channels of communication, communication strategies appropriate to the age, the features of problem-solving and problem-solving, as well as stimulating communication.
- Knows the concepts of personality, personality typologies, characteristics of mature personality, aspects of self-knowledge and self-assessment, the basics of health psychology, the psychological foundations of the various stages of life, the kinds and causes of conflicts.
- Comprehensively understands the areas of study, methods of psychology, the most important trends in psychology, their sciences and their basic problems.
- Knows in detail the principles, the characteristics, the intervention levels of the therapist, the contexts of the nursing and patient management process, the theoretical

bases and forms of patient guidance, the levels, skills and strategies of paramedical counseling, the possibilities of continuous and deliberate development of personality and professional competence

- Familiar with the ethical concepts, the ethical health care features, ethical problems occurring in the health system and their potential solutions and alternatives in the domestic context.
- Familiar with the legal concepts, the characteristics of legitimate patient care, the main legal problems in the health system and their potential solutions, alternatives in the health system, and the rights and obligations of clients and care providers.
- Widely acquainted with the legal concepts, the characteristics of legitimate patient care, the main legal problems in the health system and their potential solutions, alternatives in the health system, and the rights and obligations of clients and care providers.
- Knows in detail the demographic basics indicators, the epidemiological indicators of the population's health status, the frequency, risk factors, the public health aspirations, the fields of activity, sociological, health sociological and cultural theories and approaches of the main public diseases, and knows the sociological and health sociological approach to health preservation and development.
- Familiar with the various forms of social care and the current policy of social care.
- Knows the psychic and physical basics of addictions, the most common types of addictions, the significance of self-help programs and groups

<u>b) abilities</u>

- Capable of detecting health-damaging factors, separating physiological and abnormalities from one another, taking steps appropriate to the level of competence, or suggesting a solution.
- Applies your knowledge of typical pathological defects and changes in practical work.
- Applies knowledge of typical pathological defects and changes in your practical work
- Being able to understand the relationships between pharmacy, clinic, diagnostics and therapy in the course of the patient's care and, in the knowledge of these, is able to fulfill his duties as a specialist in the field of specialization.
- Able to properly integrate biophysical and healthcare technical skills into its practical activities and to be able to apply them when using diagnostic test procedures and therapeutic tools.
- Capable of performing workflows as well as the ability to fulfill hygiene needs (the tools, procedures and tools used in the institution) to comply with the rules of asepsis antisepsis and nosocomial surveillance criteria and the rules for separate collection of waste.
- Able to choose the appropriate bed type, bed position, posture, comfort, patient mobility and mobilization tools, procedures and procedures.
- Able to evaluate the results obtained independently of the observation of vital parameters (including mantle and core temperature, facial types, respiration pattern types, pulse rate and qualities, pulse rate, noninvasive blood pressure measurement).
- Able to carry out physical pacing.
- Able to assess pain and apply physical pain relief procedures.
- Capable of conducting professional communication tailored to the partner, both oral and written, communicating effectively with the patient, the family, the community

and the ability to build trust with the patient, family and community through interpersonal skills.

- Being able to use the necessary psychological basis for the pursuit of a psycho-somatic approach in practicing his profession is able to adequately treat the problems of interpersonal relationships between the patient and the healthcare professional, to recognize and treat basic psychological characteristics of the patient.

- Able to see the system of legal sources that regulate health care, the rules of their application, and apply the relevant legal terminology correctly, inform clients about patient rights and the possibilities to enforce them according to their competence limits.

- Able to assess the health status of the population and define priorities at individual and community levels and be able to plan and implement effective interventions.

- Depending on its field of activity, it can actively contribute to the resolution of public health issues, the organization and implementation of screening tests, and the development and application of health promotion materials.

- Can prepare a personal health plan, provide health counseling, and collaborate effectively with team members to improve the health of the community.

- Identifies and adequately integrates the patient with addiction in the care system and is able to isolate and recognize the risk and protective factors involved in the development of addictive behavior, recognize deviant behavior and guide the patient to the appropriate care system.

- Able to perform client training and non-invasive application tasks related to the indication, action mechanism and side effects of the drug groups used.

- Able to choose and apply the pedagogical knowledge, methods and capabilities associated with his / her field of expertise to perform individual and group client and patient education tasks in accordance with client age, social status, mental and emotional ability and illness.

- Able to contribute to the performance and presentation of evidence-based research based on evidence-based research methodology and biostatistics based on the results of relevant domestic and international researches.

- Able to apply the device-free and sometimes instrumental interventions that can save the patient's injured lives in the event of sudden health damage.

- Provides cost-sensitive choices and optimum use of human resources in its activities.

- Being able to be an effective midfielder to contribute effectively to organizing tasks.

- Able to perform its work based on the principles of the quality system taking into account the principles and practical aspects of evidence-based care, and to apply the different methods and tools in a coordinated manner to improve the quality

- Possesses microbiological knowledge of recognizing and preventing infectious diseases and epidemics. Being able to observe and obey your work

D. Special skills and knowledge of Paramedics

a) knowledge

- Familiar with the organizational structure and institutional system of domestic healthcare, including the location, role and relationship of emergency care and emergency care.

- Familiar with the organization and operation of the rescue service in Hungary, the rules of service, operation and behavior of operational rescue work.

- Familiar with the institutional role, framework, organization and tasks of hospital emergency care, the relevant legislation, the rules of operation and behavior of hospital care.

- Familiar with modern tools, medicines, bandages and instruments used for pre-hospital and hospital care and emergency care, and their safe use.
- Familiarizes with the pathological basis, pathology, diagnostic options, treatment options and alternatives of current treatment requiring emergency care.
- Knows the recommendations and protocols relevant to domestic and international
- Familiar with the relevant legislation in the field of pre-hospital and hospital emergency care, with particular reference to patient rights and its limitations.

<u>b) abilities</u>

- Able to set up, professionally and safely implement the interventions necessary for the emergence of urgent patient care, to prevent, detect and mitigate the undesirable consequences.
- Able to apply the acquired knowledge properly in all urgent cases on site and in emergency medical care within medical facilities.
- Capable of triage activity related to patient-related professional protocols.
- Able to perform emergency and organizational tasks within the competence of major accidents and illnesses or disaster sites.
- Capable of starting the treatment of a poisoned patient, creating a safe environment for the patient, initiating decontamination and organizing the patient's definitive care
- Conducts complication-free delivery, recognizes complications, and minimizes their consequences.
- Provides the neonate professionally, eliminates emergencies around-birth and birth.
- Capable of organizing, managing, evaluating and correcting the work of a patient care team.
- Capable of training first aid, attending training and retraining of rescue and rescue drivers, and holding first-aid courses in appropriate educational establishments.

- Able to be a member of the hospital acute supply team in accordance with the competence of hospitals for urgent care.
- Able to independently develop its knowledge and problem-solving skills, access literature, draw the right scientific conclusions, and apply current scientific results in patient care.
- Establishes a "death sentence", recognizes the circumstances of natural and extraordinary death and initiates further action if necessary.
- Provides and maintains the interoperability of the airway by means of anchoring and auxiliary devices, assisted breathing assisted or controlled by a controlled manner, independently selecting the appropriate ventilation mode.
- Performs a defined level of procedural pick-up and, if necessary, elevated level of air travel along the current valid protocols.
- Recognizes and eliminates cardiac arrhythmia by means of medicated electrical intervention (cardioversion, defibrillation), where appropriate, the replacement of spontaneous stimulation by a transtatic non-invasive pacemaker, independently recognizes the indications of cardiological intervention interventions, the related pathway management tasks, the patient's definitive care team, working according to protocols.
- Ensures the correct blood flow, oxygen and nutrient supply of the tissues, decides independently about the interventions that provide it, and then executes them
- Recognizes the pathologies of the central and peripheral nervous system independently, takes responsibility for the pathology of the patient, endangers life threatening and sustained tissue damage by carrying out self-selected interventions
- Measures and recognizes the environmental hazards, protects the patient, himself and the members of the patient care team, minimizing the effects on him.

- Independently able to create group diagnosis for emergency care.

  For this reason, the scope of the instruments without the need for an emergency tool (such as invasive, laboratory and imaging) is set up, professionally executed or performed, independently evaluated and interpreted the findings of the investigations and synthesizes the results.

- Recognizing the limitations of the possibilities or abilities of a therapist, consulted by a professional manager, a physician or a specialist, in the framework of cooperation, interprets and implements the results of the consultation.

- His intervention succeeds in recognizing the limitations of failure due to the characteristic features of emergency care, in response to a self-determined choice of alternative available patient care options.

- Responsible for recognizing the condition of the patient, preventing the deterioration of the condition. To this end, it decides on the necessary method and extent of patient monitoring, monitoring, and the scope of the necessary tests.

- Observes the illness and consciousness of the patient, the airway (potentially endangering its permeability), respiratory rate, respiration depth and respiration pattern, patient's skin and mucous membranes.

- Prepares an electrocardiogram (ECG) and evaluates it independently.

- Regularly measures or measures the patient's oxygen saturation, end-of-life carbon dioxide (EtCO2), arterial blood pressure, pulse rate and heart rate, blood glucose, body mantle and core temperature.

- Independently evaluates the outcome of the arterial blood gas test, the need for correction and its extent.

- Determines how to determine the patient's state of consciousness, arterial pressure, the intensity of the patient's pain, the amount of fluid intake and drainage.

- Interventions in self-selected therapy in the course of the pathology of the emergency care field.
- Provides and maintains an airway with supra- and infraglottic means, where appropriate with the implementation of congestion.
- Performs the deterioration of the breast cavity and the pericardium in order to prevent or prevent the onset of life, and perform thoracic drainage and thoracostomy.
- Replaces fluid, electrolyte, intravenous (peripheral venous or, in specially justified cases, central venous) or intravenously.
- Recognizes signs of sepsis, severe sepsis and septic shock, begins patient fluid therapy, suspected meningococcal disease, and provides antibiotic prophylaxis for members of the supplying team.
- Gives or dispenses a medication via the enteric and parenteral route according to valid professional protocols.
- Reduces pain with psychic driving, medication, cold, warm therapy, by choosing or promoting optimal position (positioning).
- Performs appropriate physical and instrumental tests, uses bedside diagnosis, evaluates data obtained during the exercise, self-exercises the competencies specified in the pre-hospital care, carries out specific interventions under the supervision of the shift supervisor, such as: provision of an intraosseal-pathway, wound supply and plaster installation.
- Mitigates the pain pharmaceutically, firmly attenuated and the patient is taken.
- Stimulates, limbs, spine, starts optimizing circulating blood volume, prevents the patient from overheating, overheating, minimizing the formation of acidosis caused by tissue blood flow, attaching injuries to the injuries, ensuring compliance with the rules of asepsis and antisepsis, and the patient's integrity of the patient supplying team

- Selects his injured body position.
- Provides effective pain relief and proper fluid replacement.
- By catheter, he ensures unhindered discharge of urine.

c) Attitude

- Open and susceptible to knowing and applying scientifically proven professional basics of health and medicine.
- Initiates and accepts team-based patient care, recognizes the values of collective work, demands criticism of its decisions, and seeks out consultative decision-making.
- Open to professional consultation, initiates communication with patients, evaluates its results and is open to accommodating the alternative.
- Demands professional development, is open to accepting new scientific achievements, seeks to get to know them.
- Relates to the sick person with empathy, considers communication important, recognizes the patient's needs and needs.
- Committed to quality patient care, his / her own work and colleagues' work in justified cases, in order to comply with this.
- Undertakes public awareness, health promotion, and patient information.

d) autonomy and responsibility

- Immediately intervenes in the pathologies directly or indirectly endangering the patient's life, recognizing them without delay, in which they perform lifesaving interventions, taking into account the age-specific features.
- Performs complex resuscitation (ALS), leading as unit leader.
- Treats the injured person, self-guided, the damaged body area is correctly recorded and immobilized.

- Provides the burning patient independently: it determines the extent and severity of combustion.
- Airways burns and injured people
- Provides the burning patient independently: determines the extent and severity of combustion.
- Recognizes respiratory burns on time, provided that the patient is properly trained.
- Efforts to prevent combustion-related infections and complications.
- In toxophysiologic patient, he starts emergency treatment in accordance with toxidromas, with particular regard to decontamination, antidote use, and maintenance of vital functions.
- Responsible for keeping the patient's integrity healthy.
- Self-relieving, recognizing complications and minimizing their consequences.
- Provides the neonate professionally, eliminates emergencies around birth and birth, and, if justified, uses contraction techniques, epiziotomy.
- In the field of on-the-spot care (eg.pre-hospitally and hospitally), he / she decides on the necessity of the patient's hospital treatment, in cooperation with the shift specialist, and the further treatment in his / her home where the patient is informed in detail, and shall be responsible for the accompanying documentation.
- As in a hospital with patient in need, he is capable of performing complex resuscitation as a team member, team leader, detecting and evaluating the vital parameters of patients, making immediate decisions on the basis of available information.
- Coordinates intra- and inter-hospital transport.

As a consequence, both pre-hospitally and intra-hospitally, Paramedics are entitled and required to act according to the above described criteria. [16] Hence, the practice which still occurs in Hungary that paramedics are employed as nurses in hospitals is absolutely illegal, since according to the current Hungarian legislation, Paramedics must be employed as paramedics with the criteria mentioned and detailed in our essay.

VIII. Charts and Other Characteristics

Chart One. The rise of number of Paramedics in the past two decades

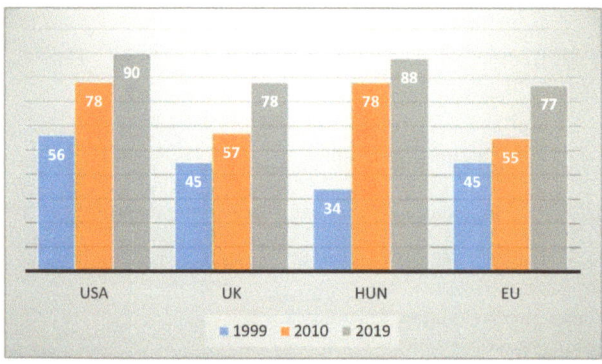

Source: www.ksh.hu

Obviously it should be noted that in Hungary there was a significant rise in number of paramedics at the end of the millennium. The reason for this is that before 1999 there was only one university in the country training paramedics, from 1999 there was another one to start the training, and from 2004 the third one came into picture. Still, there is a very low number of paramedics graduating each year in Hungary (n<50), which is not so prospective for the future. As it can be observed on the chart, the number of paramedics graduating is rising anyplace in the countries we observed, however, the most significant rise could be noted in Hungary. Unlike

---

[16] see also. https://www.ncbi.nlm.nih.gov/pubmed/20097499

in the case of nurses and medical doctors, fewer paramedics leave our country for better work possibilities.

Chart two. Paramedics leaving the country for better opportunities

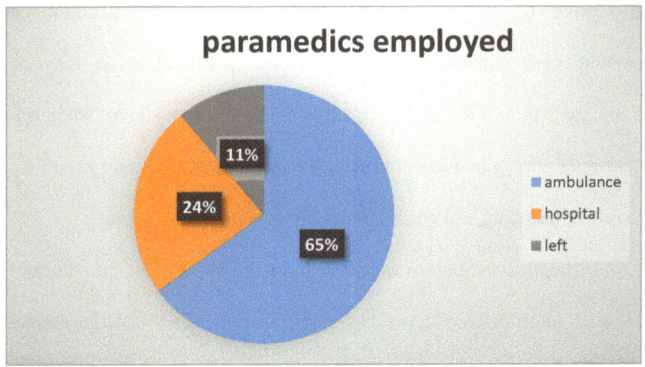

Source:

https://alfahir.hu/2018/02/15/elvandorlas_kivandorlas_nagy_britannia_nemetorszag_ausztria_ksh_nepessegtudomanyi

In Hungary, there is a very small portion of paramedics leaving the country yet. The reason for this is that Paramedics are accepted on the ambulance cars and on the emergency wards only in Anglo-Saxon countries such as Great Britain, the USA, New Zealand, Canada and Australia. Paramedic mobility, therefore, from Hungary is not that significant unlike other health care workers and medical doctors, who could be easily welcomed in German speaking countries as well. In the German system, there is not a qualification like Paramedic, hence it is very hard to adapt paramedic degrees to the German legal regulation. In Germany, Austrian and Switzerland, Sänitaters work on ambulances with different, however not that broad competencies like in Anglo-Saxon countries, it is rather similar to the competence BSc or Msc nurses. [17]

---

[17]see.https://alfahir.hu/2018/02/15/elvandorlas_kivandorlas_nagy_britannia_nemetorszag_ausztria_ksh_nepessegtudomanyi

IX. Conclusions

A career as a Paramedic or Medic can be incredibly rewarding for compassionate, courageous and driven people who want to make a difference. Patient Transport Officer, Emergency Medical Technician, Ambulance officer[18], Industrial medic, Ambulance attendant or Medic/Paramedic. They could even specialize in aeromedical paramedics or disaster management – it truly is a diverse career path. Moreover, it is especially true today, when the legal regulation allows you to take part in treating at hospitals as well as other surgery rooms.

By choosing a vocational style of learning, we can fit our study around our lifestyle.

As well as creating a future for themselves, paramedics will have the opportunity to continue in current job and earn as learn. Qualifications in pre-hospital emergency care like our means that they will be well prepared to take on the many job roles available in the private sector.

Furthermore, for the fact that paramedics typically respond to emergency situations, their ability to quickly assess a medical condition and provide the appropriate medical care can make the difference between life and death. Whilst this can be highly stressful for paramedics, they could also gain a high level of satisfaction from knowing that they play an important role in society. As a result, the career may be extremely rewarding for those who enjoy helping others in emergency.

As a conclusion, as experts in Health Care Law as well as Paramedic Studies and Practice, we could conclude that the legal regulations in the USA, the UK, Canada and in Hungary can provide a legitimate frame to utilize and employ paramedics in hospital treatment too – so they can be employed on-board (on an ambulance) and off-board (at hospitals) as well.

---

[18] in Hungary and Australia (eds.)

X. Bibliography

Books and articles

Dan Sundhal, *Portraits of an Emergency*, NY, 2006.

Dan Pronk, *Arterial Tourniquets: For Police Officers, Law Enforcement and other First-Responders,* Tacmed Australia, 2016.

Göbl G. Oxiológia, Medicina, Budapest, 2006.

Philip Allen Green, Trauma Room Two, Norton, 2015.

Jannice Hudson, *Trauma Junkie: Memoirs of an Emergency Flight Nurse*, NY, 2010.

Kevin Hazzard, *Thousand Naked Strangers: A Paramedic's Wild Ride to the Edge and Back*, NY, 2016.

Kelly Grayson, *A Paramedic's Story: Life, Death and Everything In Between*, NY, 2010.

Albert Reyes, Fresh Out from EMT School, California, 2017.

Mary Roach Stiff: *The Curious Lives of Human Cadavers*, Norton Publishing, 2003.
Dennis Smith, *Report from Engine Co. 82, NY*1999

Talabér j., "Mentő protokoll? - eljárásrend szemle jogász szemmel"., MSOTKE Konferencia, Budapest, 2015. november 12-15.

Talabér j., , Kompetenciák a sürgősségi betegellátásban , Előadás: Szeged, MRT Kongresszus, 2007. szeptember 15.

Talabér j., Az ellátók és ellátottak jogai és kötelezettségei, Pusztaföldvár, Egészség Napok Továbbképzés sorozat, 2018. május 23.

Talabér j.,Off-board mentőtiszt - jogszerűen a sürgősségin és az orvosi ügyeleten? , MSOTKE, 2018. (poszter), Siófok.

Troy Valente, *Capnography, King of the ABC's: A Systematic Approach for Paramedics*, Norton Publishing, 2010.

V.Clarke, G.Harris, S. Cowland (eds), Ethics and Laws For Paramedics, London, 2009.

Web pages visited

http://ec.europa.eu/growth/toolsdatabases/regprof/index.cfm?action=regprof&id_regprof=264 27.

https://en.wikipedia.org/wiki/Paramedics_in_the_United_States"Nationwide Directory of Paramedic Schools". Retrieved 2008-11-07.

"National EMS Scope of Practice" (PDF). Retrieved 2012-11-11.

https://www.mheducation.co.uk/openup/chapters/9780335243877.pdf.

http://www.mentomuzeum.hu/eng/about-nas.

http://statinfo.ksh.hu/Statinfo/haViewer.jsp.

www.dabasmok.hu.

see also. https://www.ncbi.nlm.nih.gov/pubmed/20097499.

see.https://alfahir.hu/2018/02/15/elvandorlas_kivandorlas_nagy_britannia_nemetorszag_ausztria_ksh_nepessegtudomanyi.

Ad Maiorem Dei Gloriam

Dr János Talabér, 2018-2019.

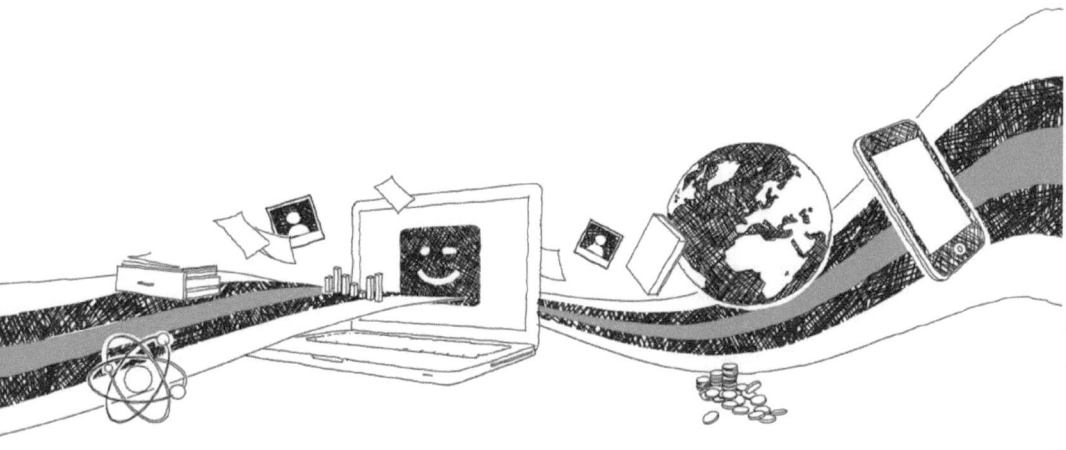
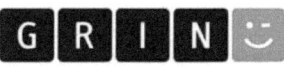